RE THIS SIMPLE TEST TO FIND OU
MORE EFFECTIVELY THAN PROZAC? IF THERE WAS A
U CALL YOUR DOCTOR IMMEDIATELY? ARE NEW SHOES
HE POWER TO MAKE YOU MORE APPEALING TO THE
RUIN YOUR FEET AND YOUR REPUTATION? DO YOU
OSS FOR A SALE ON MANOLO BLAHNIKS? WOULD YOU
O THEIR FEET? IF YOUR CLOSET WAS ON FIRE, WHICH
E YOU WORE GALOSHES? FINISH THIS VERSE: "THERE
BOCA b) A SHOE c) HOPES OF A SON-IN-LAW." WHAT
HAN THREE PAIRS OF BLACK SHOES? MORE THAN SIX?
R SHOE SIZE? WHAT IS YOUR SHOE SIZE? WHEN YOU
NE COLOR? HAVE YOU EVER RENTED A PAIR OF SHOES
UR MOTHER WEARS COMBAT BOOTS" STOP BEING AN
UR SKIRT WHEN YOU WORE YOUR PATENT LEATHER
E THE DICTATOR OF A SMALL HUMID COUNTRY, WOULD
COUP D'ÉTAT? HAVE YOU EVER SPENT MORE MONEY
CHASE PRICE? HAVE YOU EVER SPENT MORE MONEY
DUCT OF A SMALL HUMID COUNTRY? DID YOU EVER
R LOVED A PAIR OF SHOES MORE THAN LIFE ITSELF?

Nothing risqué, nothing gained.

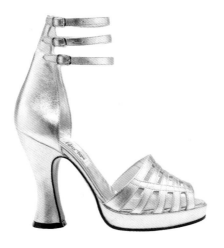

ALEXANDER WOOLLCOTT

a PASSION for SHOES

LINDA SUNSHINE
& MARY TIEGREEN

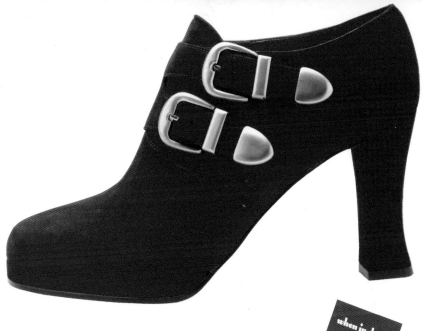

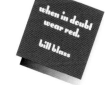

when in doubt
wear red.

bill blass

a welcome book

andrews and mcmeel
kansas city

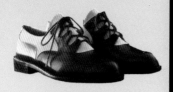

**I make love with
my feet.**

Fred Astaire

For information write:
Andrews and McMeel,
A Universal Press Syndicate Company,
4900 Main Street, Kansas City, Missouri 64112

Note: Every effort has been made to locate the copyright owners
of the material used in the book. Please let us know if an error has
been made, and we will make any necessary changes in subsequent
printings.

Credits and copyright notices appear on pages 62 and 63.

A Welcome Book
Welcome Enterprises, Inc.
575 Broadway, New York, New York 10012

Edited by Linda Sunshine
Designed by Mary Tiegreen

Library of Congress Catalog Card Number:
95-77549

ISBN: 0-8362-0799-8

Printed in China by Toppan Printing
10 9 8 7 6 5 4 3 2 1

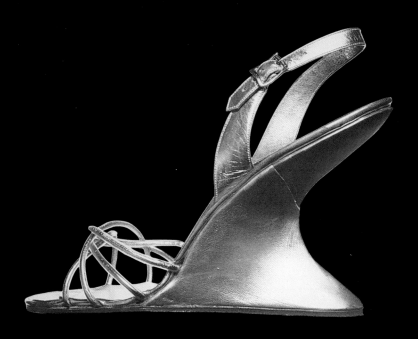

We are shaped and fashioned by what we love.

Johann Wolfgang von Goethe

Do I really need them?

I don't know. I don't really **NEED** them, but they make my feet look so elegant, so sexy, so SMALL!!! I don't know. Should I get them? Don't I have a pair just like them? No, they're not that much the same. True, they're the same color but the heel is a little different, I think. Wow, these are *really* expensive. Still, I didn't have lunch today so I saved money. Oh, **THEY LOOK REALLY GOOD FROM THE BACK.** Let me think. I may need new shoes for over the holidays for parties and stuff if I get invited to any parties—and for a morale booster in case I don't. They're *SO* **GORGEOUS,** but they are a little tight—not that tight, not like **CRIPPLING TIGHT.** I wouldn't wear them every day anyway. At parties, it's not like you have to stand around all the time; I wouldn't be walking all that much in them and look **HOW GREAT THEY LOOK WHEN I'M SITTING DOWN.** I love them; they're absolutely beautiful even though they do pinch in the toe just a little. Maybe I should try a bigger size. No, then they'll look so humongous that I might as well wear the shoe boxes. **SO WHAT'S A LITTLE PAIN?** You have to suffer to be beautiful, and it's important to treat yourself well and have some self-esteem. I deserve these shoes. I've put up with a lot this week, and no one else is going to buy them for me so I'd better take care of Numero Uno. I suppose I could ask the salesman to stretch them for me; I'll probably get **BLISTERS** the first few times I wear them. I'm used to that; I went through a whole box of Band-Aids with the last pair of shoes I bought here. Oh, who cares? They'll stretch; **SUEDE ALWAYS STRETCHES,** and it doesn't wear all that well, which makes you wonder why any sane person would spend all this money. Jeez, this is almost a week's pay; I can't afford these. This is ridiculous. **BUT I REALLY WANT THEM;** and I promise not to buy another expensive thing for the rest of the year. It's not like I'm buying roller blades or anything stupid like that magenta raincoat I bought last year and never wore. And they're not that expensive if you factor in the cost per wear and compare the price to the cost of a college education and, oh, who am I kidding? **I ABSOLUTELY CAN'T AFFORD THESE SHOES,** and even though they look fabulous, they're **NOT PRACTICAL,** and they're **TOO EXPENSIVE,** and they **DON'T FIT WELL,** and I am just going to take them off my feet and hand them back to the salesman and get the hell out of this store . . .

"Sir? I'll take these.
And do they also come in **red**?"

He sat bowed over, his head between his hands, staring at the hearthrug, and at the tip of the satin shoe that showed under her dress. Suddenly he knelt down and kissed the shoe. ❦

Edith Wharton
THE AGE OF INNOCENCE

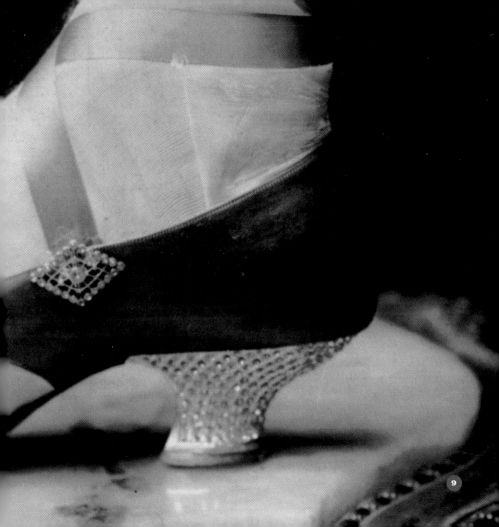

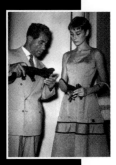

I have divided the women who have come to me into three categories; the Cinderella, the Venus, and the Aristocrat. The Cinderella takes a shoe smaller than size six, the Venus takes size six, the Aristocrat takes a seven or larger.

VENUS IS USUALLY OF GREAT BEAUTY, GLAMOUR, AND SOPHISTICATION, YET UNDER HER GLITTERING EXTERIOR SHE IS OFTEN ESSENTIALLY A HOMEBODY LOVING THE SIMPLE THINGS OF LIFE.

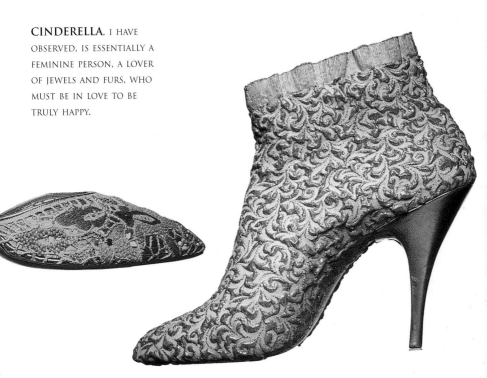

CINDERELLA, I HAVE OBSERVED, IS ESSENTIALLY A FEMININE PERSON, A LOVER OF JEWELS AND FURS, WHO MUST BE IN LOVE TO BE TRULY HAPPY.

ARISTOCRATS ARE SENSITIVE, EVEN MOODY, BUT POSSESS A GREAT DEPTH OF UNDERSTANDING.

SALVATORE FERRAGAMO

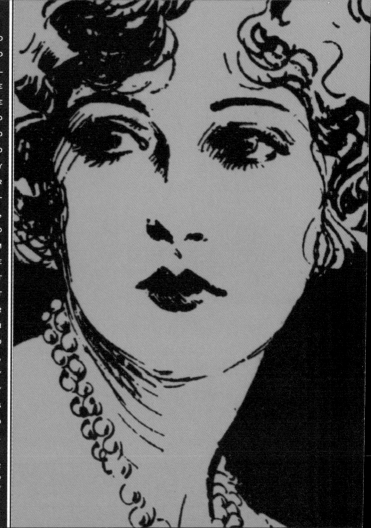

ANNABEL AND MIDGE DID, AND COMPLETELY, ALL THAT YOUNG OFFICE WORKERS ARE BESOUGHT NOT TO DO. THEY PAINTED THEIR LIPS AND THEIR NAILS, THEY DARKENED THEIR LASHES AND LIGHTENED THEIR HAIR, AND SCENT SEEMED TO SHIMMER FROM THEM. THEY WORE THIN, BRIGHT DRESSES, TIGHT OVER THEIR BREASTS AND HIGH ON THEIR LEGS, AND TILTED SLIPPERS, FANCIFULLY STRAPPED. THEY LOOKED CONSPICUOUS AND CHEAP AND CHARMING.

DOROTHY PARKER
"THE STANDARD
OF LIVING"

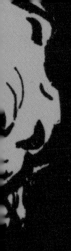

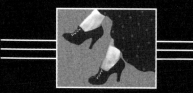

HAZEL MORSE WAS A LARGE, FAIR WOMAN OF THE TYPE THAT INCITES SOME MEN WHEN THEY USE THE WORD "BLONDE" TO CLICK THEIR TONGUES AND WAG THEIR HEADS ROGUISHLY. SHE PRIDED HERSELF UPON HER SMALL FEET AND SUFFERED FOR HER VANITY, BOXING THEM IN SNUB-TOED, HIGH-HEELED SLIPPERS OF THE SHORTEST BEARABLE SIZE.

DOROTHY PARKER
"BIG BLONDE"

Brooke Shields

BY GEORGIA DULLEA

PITTSBURGH, NOVEMBER 10, 1994. THE MORNING AFTER HER OPENING NIGHT HERE IN THE ROAD SHOW OF "GREASE!" FINDS BROOKE SHIELDS PADDING AROUND HER HOTEL SUITE IN BARE FEET, WHICH, THANKS TO BUNION SURGERY, ARE NOW AS LOVELY AS THE REST OF HER. "I HAD TO HAVE BOTH FEET BROKEN," SHE SAYS, WINCING, "BUT NOW I CAN WEAR HIGH HEELS WITHOUT THREE TYLENOLS." —*THE NEW YORK TIMES*

WHILE JOE WAS NO STRANGER TO SHOPPING FOR SHOES, HE WAS AWARE THAT SHOPPING FOR WOMEN'S SHOES WAS ANOTHER UPHEAVAL ENTIRELY. JOE'S MOTHER, AS FAR AS HE KNEW, HAD NEVER PURCHASED A COMFORTABLE, WELL-FITTING PAIR OF SHOES. IF THE SHOES WERE COMFORTABLE, THEY WOULD UNDOUBTEDLY BE UGLY, ORTHOPEDIC IN SOME WAY. WOMEN SUFFERED FOR THEIR SHOES. WOMEN'S SHOES WERE DESIGNED TO BE ANTITHETICAL TO WALKING, LET ALONE WALKING BRISKLY. AS A CHILD, JOE HAD ONCE STEPPED INTO A PAIR OF HIS MOTHER'S HIGH HEELS. AT FIRST HE HAD WELCOMED THE ADDITIONAL ELEVATION, BUT THEN HE HAD EXPERIENCED ONLY TORTURE, VIA SHOOTING PAINS IN HIS SHINS. ALL OF FEMINISM, JOE KNEW, COULD BE ENCAPSULATED IN WOMEN'S STRUGGLE TO FORSAKE THE SPIKE HEEL.

Paul Rudnick, *I'll Take It*

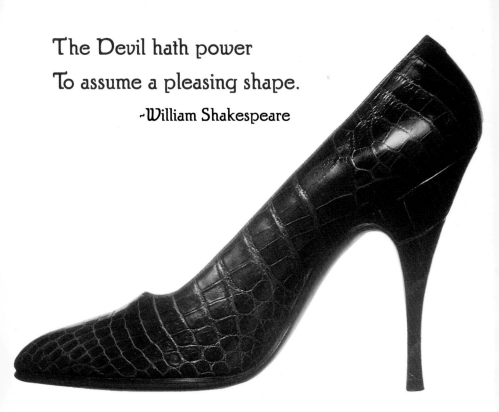

The Devil hath power
To assume a pleasing shape.

~William Shakespeare

Ferragamo Court Shoe 1958-59

THIS SIMPLE, EXTREMELY ELEGANT SHOE WAS DESIGNED FOR MARILYN MONROE. A PAIR OF FERRAGAMO SHOES BELONGING TO THE
ACTRESS WERE SOLD AT A SOTHEBY'S AUCTION FOR MANY THOUSANDS OF DOLLARS.

THE ANSWER TO THE SOUL SEARCHING QUESTION "WHO AM I?" IS AS CLOSE AS YOUR CLOSET FLOOR~

YOU ARE YOUR SHOES!

LISTEN TO THE SOLEFUL STATEMENTS OF YOUR FOOTWEAR:

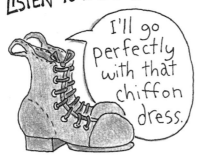

COMBAT CROSSOVER

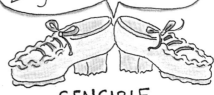

SENSIBLE

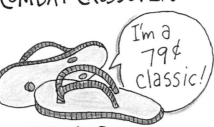

FLIP FLOP

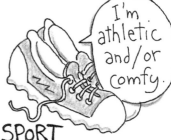

SPORT

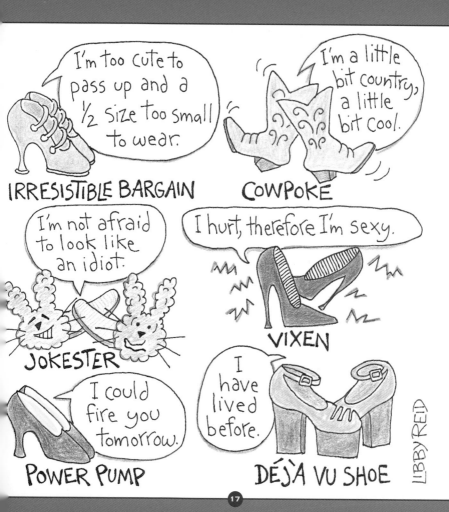

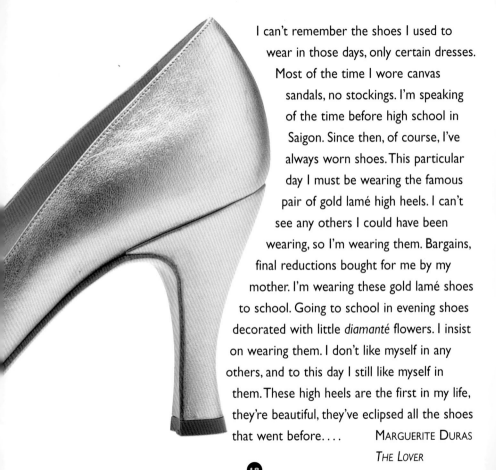

I can't remember the shoes I used to wear in those days, only certain dresses. Most of the time I wore canvas sandals, no stockings. I'm speaking of the time before high school in Saigon. Since then, of course, I've always worn shoes. This particular day I must be wearing the famous pair of gold lamé high heels. I can't see any others I could have been wearing, so I'm wearing them. Bargains, final reductions bought for me by my mother. I'm wearing these gold lamé shoes to school. Going to school in evening shoes decorated with little *diamanté* flowers. I insist on wearing them. I don't like myself in any others, and to this day I still like myself in them. These high heels are the first in my life, they're beautiful, they've eclipsed all the shoes that went before. . . .

MARGUERITE DURAS
THE LOVER

18

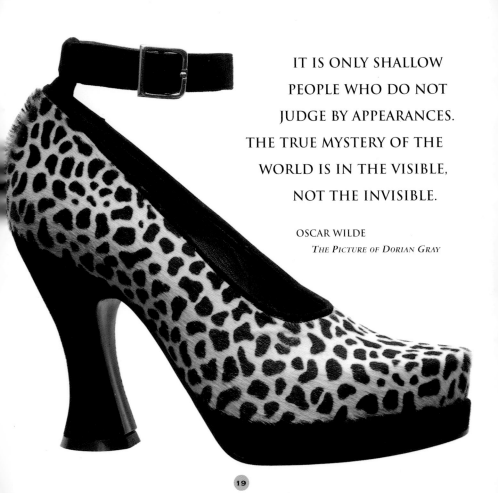

IT IS ONLY SHALLOW
PEOPLE WHO DO NOT
JUDGE BY APPEARANCES.
THE TRUE MYSTERY OF THE
WORLD IS IN THE VISIBLE,
NOT THE INVISIBLE.

OSCAR WILDE
THE PICTURE OF DORIAN GRAY

I like shoes that make your feet look cute, like puppy paws. And high heels if they make your legs look long. A guy once told me I had long legs; so I capitalized on them by wearing high heels. Unfortunately, I have a small head . . . the longer I make my legs, the smaller my head looks.

Gilda Radner
Cheap Chic Update

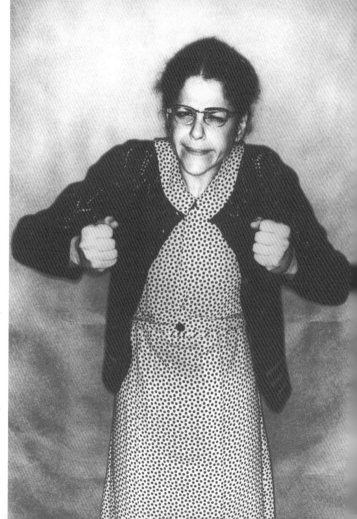

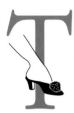The realization hit me heavily, like a .44 Magnum smashing into my skull. . . . Dating. I will have to start dating again. Please, God, no, don't make me do it! . . . I'll need new dresses, new jewelry, new sweaters, trousers, underwear. And shoes! Shoes tell everything, shoes have to be perfect! Men like high heels, right? I can't walk in high heels. Well, I can try. For a really important date, I can just see myself spending $250 on a pair of drop-dead heels. This time will be different, I tell myself, this time I will be able to walk. But after an hour the ball of my foot will cramp up. I know it, and I'll hobble. **"Is anything wrong?" he'll ask me solicitously, "you're limping."** And I won't know where to look. I won't be able to say, "These fucking shoes are crippling me and if I don't take them off this minute I'll be maimed for life!" Because then he'll know I just bought them, that I bought them to go out on a date with him. And that will make him feel weird and pressured to know that this date was a big deal for me and he'll realize that I'm not as popular and sophisticated as he thought I was if I had to buy a special pair of shoes that I can't even walk in for chrissakes just for a date with him. So I have to explain the limping in such a way that it won't have to do with shoes. An old war wound?

Cynthia Heimel
A Girl's Guide to Chaos

SHOES ARE THE

EXCLAMATION

POINT AT THE

END OF THE

FASHION

STATEMENT.

⚜

LAURIE

SCHECTER

INTERVIEW

Attractive Styles for Attracting Dates

FLATTERING FOOTWEAR IS THE FIRST STEP TOWARD AN ACTIVE SOCIAL LIFE

Your phone will start ringing off the hook once you slip into our high-quality fancy footwear. All of our shoes are styled to attract that special someone and increase your dating pleasure.

A SADDLE OXFORDS
Smart, comfortable, an all-time favorite for sport, casual, or campus wear. So clean cut, these rah-rah saddle shoes will even make the town tramp look like a cheerleader. *State width and size.* 24A4749. $4.25

B PENNY LOAFER
Popular moc-toe lounger you'll wear with all your favorite sport togs. So comfortable to slip on and off. Available in dime, nickel and quarter sizes. *State size.* 24A4754. $4.50

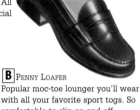

C MARY JANES
Beautifully styled with classic simplicity, these boy-pleasers are eye-catching in shiny Patent Leather. Special matte laminate guards against reflection from white underwear. *State size.* 24A4750 -Black Patent. $4.50

D SPECTATOR PUMPS
Saucy, toe-flattering date-goers feel as good as they look! Slimming 4-inch heels create sexy illusion of longer legs and thinner thighs. Not recommended for first dates, blind dates, or short dates. *State size.* 24A2082. $6.85

E DON'S BOWLING SHOES
Turn heads in your local alley with these multi-colored classics. Previously worn in league tournaments across the country. Recommended by professional bowlers. Rubber heels, smoked Elk uppers and plastic sliding left sole. For right-handed bowlers only. *State average bowling score.* 24A2077. $6.85

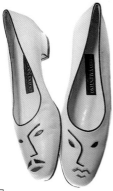

F SOPHISTICATED PUMPS
When ordinary pumps just won't do. Our fabulous guy and gal vamps are available with Caucasian, Hispanic, African-American or Oriental features! *(Gay and lesbian pairs can be special ordered.)* State size. 24A4722. Leather. $6.50

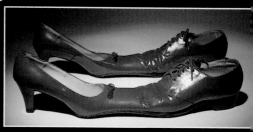

H DANCE-INSTRUCTION SHOES
First shown in the brilliant Philippa Garner's *Better Living Catalog*, here's a foolproof method for learning even the most complex steps. You dance as well as your partner immediately, regardless of previous experience or sense of rhythm. If it's the first time on the floor for both partners, you learn together, at the same pace, so interest is maintained. *State both sizes.* 24A4752 -Brown Leather $9.50

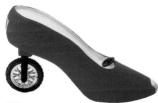

G HEELS ON WHEELS
For the gal on the go, here's the perfect shoe for getting around town in a hurry. Each pair gets at least 100 miles to the gallon. Can be reheeled at your local gas station. *Available with airbags.* 24A4731. $4.50

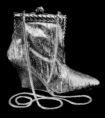

I ENCHANTED EVENING SHOEBAG
Those special nights just got specialer! Our original gold lamé shoe/bag is as practical as it is beautiful. *Put your money where your lipstick is!* 24A4731 -Lamé. $6.50

J SHE SELLS SEASHELLS
Walk the beach in style in these unique high heel seashell pumps which bring out the mermaid in all of us. *Available in fresh and saltwater species.* 24A4731. $7.50

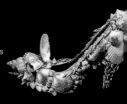

LOVE OF SHOE

Oh love of shoe. He have love of shoe. White Bucks. Black Pumps. Shoes for peace. Shoes for industry.

He watch shoe of women walking to work. He love the secretary shoe. The shoe have the good sense. It bet on Native Dancer. It play the shoe horn. The shoe be no-nonsense.

He love the no-nonsense shoe. It know when to put the foot down. It be up-front. It stand on own two feet. It wear the eyeglasses and go to Vassar on scholarship.

No-nonsense shoe have the degree in art history and work in the insurance agency. Oh he want to free her to dance the light fantastic. He want to show her the Tintoretto.

Oh the shoe. The love of shoe that stumble when she hurt when she lose the dream. She want the rhinestone clip-ons and the spike heel. She want the staccato of her heel in the spanish cabaret, the taffeta skirt at the ankle, the eye on the foot.

Yes. Yes.

Yes.

LAUREL ANN BOGEN
The Projects

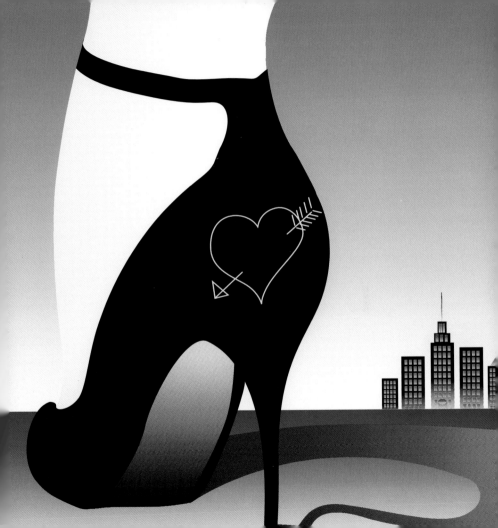

put on your dancing shoes!
turn up the heat!
it's time to
rhumba!

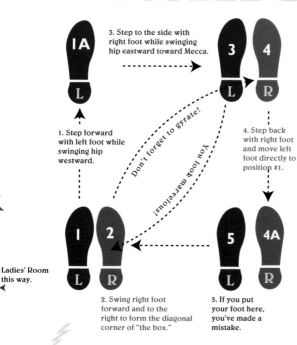

1A L

3. Step to the side with right foot while swinging hip eastward toward Mecca.

3 L **4** R

1. Step forward with left foot while swinging hip westward.

Don't forget to gyrate!

You look marvelous!

4. Step back with right foot and move left foot directly to position #1.

1 L **2** R

5 L **4A** R

Ladies' Room this way. ◄

2. Swing right foot forward and to the right to form the diagonal corner of "the box."

5. If you put your foot here, you've made a mistake.

RECOMMENDED RHUMBA SHOES*

the ricardo

evening in rio

the fernando

la bimba

*Approved by The American Salsa Association

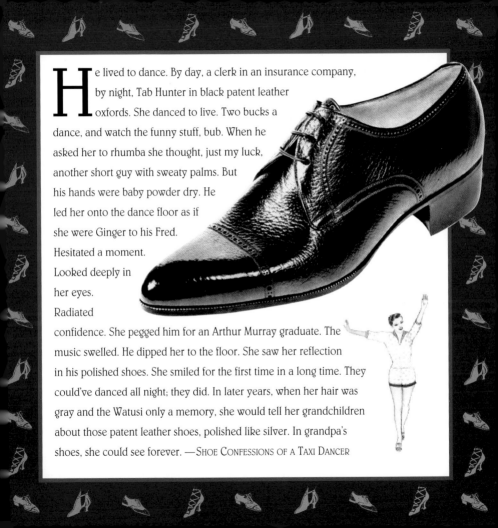

He lived to dance. By day, a clerk in an insurance company, by night, Tab Hunter in black patent leather oxfords. She danced to live. Two bucks a dance, and watch the funny stuff, bub. When he asked her to rhumba she thought, just my luck, another short guy with sweaty palms. But his hands were baby powder dry. He led her onto the dance floor as if she were Ginger to his Fred. Hesitated a moment. Looked deeply in her eyes. Radiated confidence. She pegged him for an Arthur Murray graduate. The music swelled. He dipped her to the floor. She saw her reflection in his polished shoes. She smiled for the first time in a long time. They could've danced all night; they did. In later years, when her hair was gray and the Watusi only a memory, she would tell her grandchildren about those patent leather shoes, polished like silver. In grandpa's shoes, she could see forever. —SHOE CONFESSIONS OF A TAXI DANCER

a quintessential human paradox

An air of imminent apocalypse hung over the shoe department like a wet tarpaulin as Carmen Pinchuck handed his box to Blanche Mandlestam and said, "I'd like to return these loafers. They're too small."

"Do you have a sales slip?" Blanche countered, trying to remain poised, although she confessed later that her world had suddenly begun falling apart. ("I can't deal with people since the accident," she has told friends. Six months ago, while playing tennis, she swallowed one of the balls. Since then her breathing has become irregular.)

"Er, no," Pinchuck replied nervously. "I lost it." (The central problem of his life is that he is always misplacing things. Once he went to sleep and when he awoke the bed was missing.) Now, as customers lined up behind him impatiently, he broke into a cold sweat.

"You'll have to have it O.K.'d by the floor manager," Blanche said, referring Pinchuck to Mr. Dubinsky, whom she had been having an affair

His socks compelled one's attention
without losing one's respect . . .
Saki, "Minister of Grace"

with since Halloween. (Lou Dubinsky, a
graduate of the best typing school in Europe,
was a genius until alcohol reduced his word
speed to one word per day and he was forced to
go to work in a department store.)

"Have you worn them?" Blanche continued,
fighting back tears. The notion of Pinchuk in his
loafers was unbearable to her. "My father used to wear
loafers," she confessed. "Both on the same foot."

Pinchuk was writhing now. "No," he said. "Er—I
mean yes. I had them on briefly, but only while I took a bath."

"Why did you buy them if they were too small?" Blanche asked,
unaware that she was articulating a quintessential human paradox.

Woody Allen
By Destiny Denied

HE'S A SHOE SALESMAN.

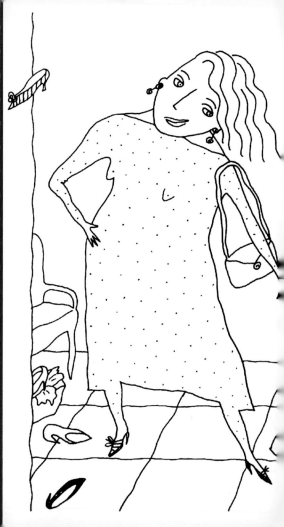

He knows that a survey of women not long ago found that more than 80% wore shoes that were at least a size too small. . . .

He knows that size fluctuates from make to make. . . . He knows that everyone has one foot that is larger than the other. . . . He knows that feet widen with age. . . . On an average day, he sells 30 to 35 pairs; when the store is really humming, put him down for 60. Working six days a week, he earns roughly $35,000 a year. Constantly upright, he knows he has to wear something soothing. He favors a Rockport wingtip in a 9½ D.

"If the Shoe Fits, Sell It
(and Another Pair)"
by N.R. Kleinfield
The New York Times

Shoes are the one thing i can buy
to wear that will still fit even though
i've gained 10 pounds.

And it doesn't matter that i haven't
been to the gym in three months
and my body is all flabby,

shoes always
look
great.

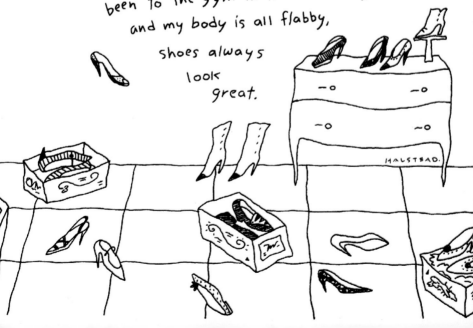

HALSTEAD.

THE "FOOT" MEASURE-
MENT WAS DEVELOPED IN
1320 IN ENGLAND BY
EDWARD II WHOSE FOOT
MEASURED 36 BARLEY
CORNS. EACH CORN WAS
ONE THIRD OF AN INCH,
WHICH ADDED UP TO
12 INCHES, OR
ONE FOOT.

JAMES SMITH, FOUNDER
OF JAMES SOUTHALL &
CO. OF NORWICH,
ENGLAND, INTRODUCED
SHOE SIZES IN 1792.

IT WAS ABOUT THE TIME
OF THE AMERICAN
CIVIL WAR THAT
MANUFACTURERS BEGAN
MAKING LEFT AND
RIGHT SHOES.

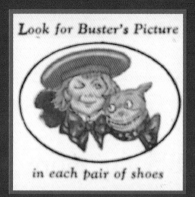

Look for Buster's Picture

in each pair of shoes

*B*oth my sister and I got one
pair of "school" and one pair of
"dress" shoes each year. We always
waited until the second week of
school in the fall to see what the
other kids were wearing. I guess
this was our follow-the-crowd
phase. Actually, the shoes always
turned out to be Buster Brown
oxfords anyway.

Annette Swanberg
from *What We Wore*
by Ellen Melinkoff

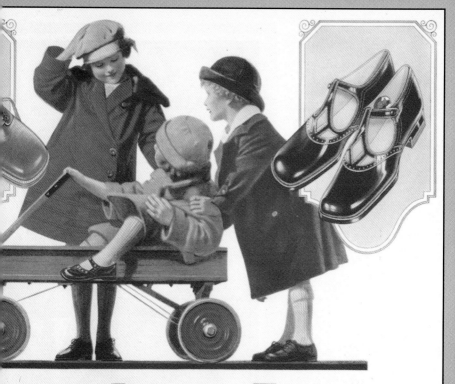

STER BROWN SHOES

> # Shoes are the first adult machines we are given to master.
>
> ## Nicholas Baker,
> ### *The Mezzanine*

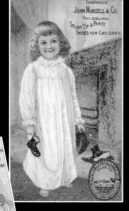

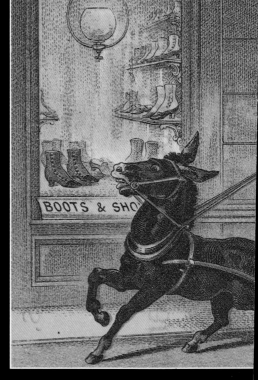

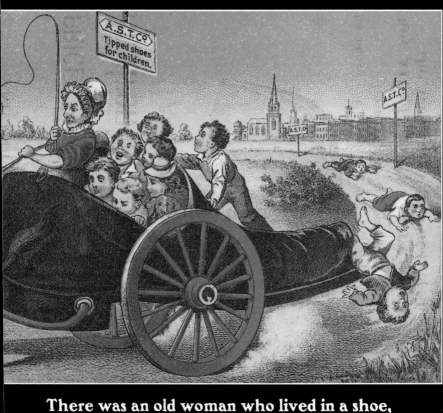

**There was an old woman who lived in a shoe,
She had so many children she didn't know what to do!**

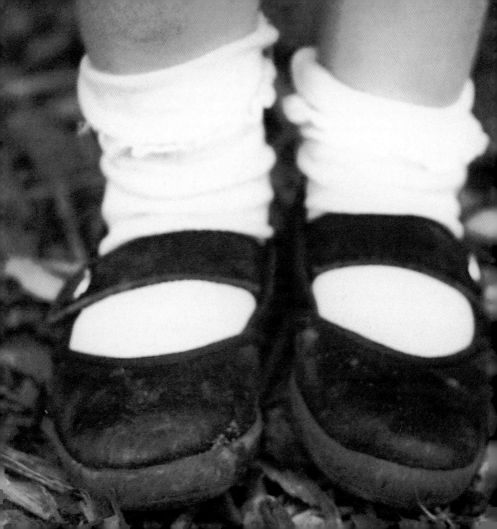

A Doll's Shoe

I had just got a new Skipper doll—to cheer me up, because my father had been in the hospital. I'd taken the doll outside and lost her shoe. My mother had spent an hour on her hands and knees, helping me search for that shoe in the thick grass. My mother—who, I always believed, could do anything—found it.

I always tell that story with affection, but I have always made fun of my mother a little for that, too. What a lot of fuss to make over something so small, I have thought to myself.

Only the fuss was about something besides a doll's shoe, of course. It was about loss and pain. Small pain, minor loss, in the scale of things. The kind of pain a mother can still control, can still prevent, maybe. Knowing, all the while, how many other sorrows there will be that she can't do anything about: Little girls who don't come to her party. Children on the playground who make fun of her overalls. Boys who ask someone else to the dance instead. Colleges she won't get into. A lover who leaves.

Joyce Maynard
Domestic Affairs

At this time the Queen was taking a journey through the country and she had her little daughter the Princess with her. The people crowded round the palace where they were staying to see them. The little Princess stood at the window to show herself. She wore neither a train nor a golden crown, but she was dressed all in white with a beautiful pair of red morocco shoes. Nothing in the world could be compared to these red shoes.

Hans Christian Anderson
THE RED SHOES

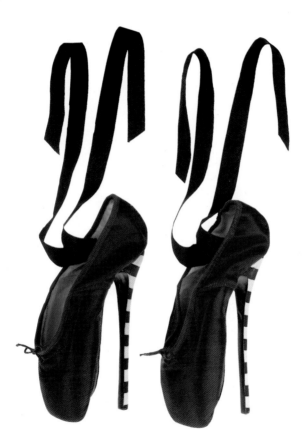

I NEED TO LIVE IN NEW SHOES.
—HEATHER WATTS, PRIMA BALLERINA

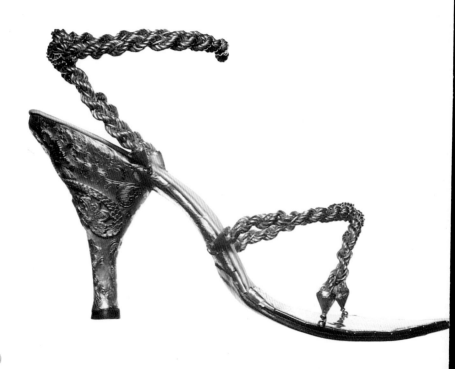

THE SHOE THAT FITS ONE PERSON PINCHES ANOTHER:

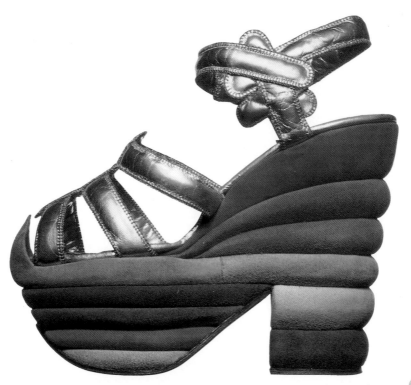

41

THERE IS NO RECIPE FOR LIVING THAT SUITS ALL CASES . . .
—CARL GUSTAV JUNG

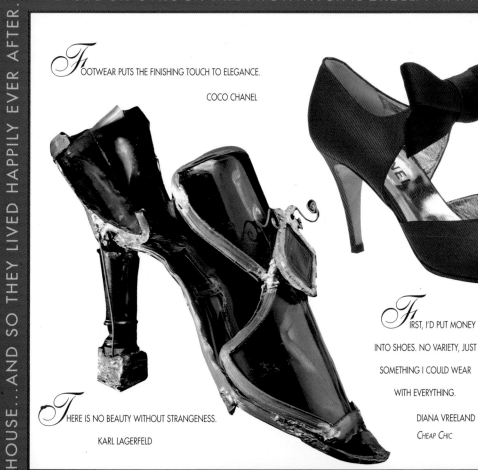

ℱOOTWEAR PUTS THE FINISHING TOUCH TO ELEGANCE.

COCO CHANEL

ℱIRST, I'D PUT MONEY
INTO SHOES. NO VARIETY, JUST
SOMETHING I COULD WEAR
WITH EVERYTHING.

DIANA VREELAND
CHEAP CHIC

ℱHERE IS NO BEAUTY WITHOUT STRANGENESS.

KARL LAGERFELD

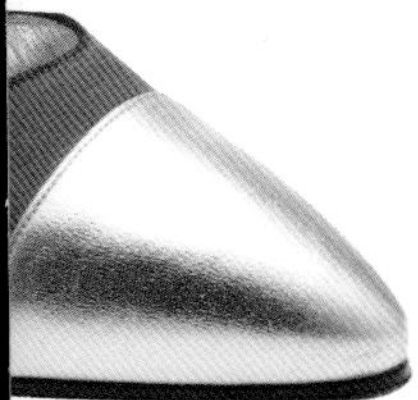

*A*T THIS MOMENT I OWN THREE PAIRS OF PLAIN BLACK LEATHER PUMPS THAT ALTERNATE ALL WINTER, SOME BLACK BEADED EVENING SLIPPERS, ONE PAIR OF FLATS. IN SUMMER I SWITCH AROUND THREE PAIRS OF BLACK PATENT AND ONE PAIR OF BONE PUMPS. FINISH.

THE CHEAPER THE SHOE, THE SIMPLER THE CUT SHOULD BE. (I CAN'T STAND PIPPY-POO THINGS ON ANY SHOES.)

... AND NO WHITE SHOES WITH DARK DRESSES. OKAY?

HELEN GURLEY BROWN

Sex and the Single Girl

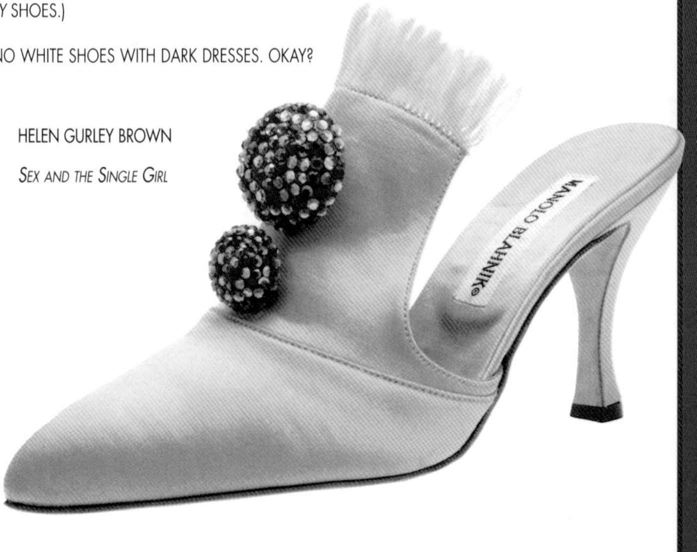

*A*DORNMENT IS NEVER ANYTHING EXCEPT A REFLECTION OF THE HEART.

COCO CHANEL

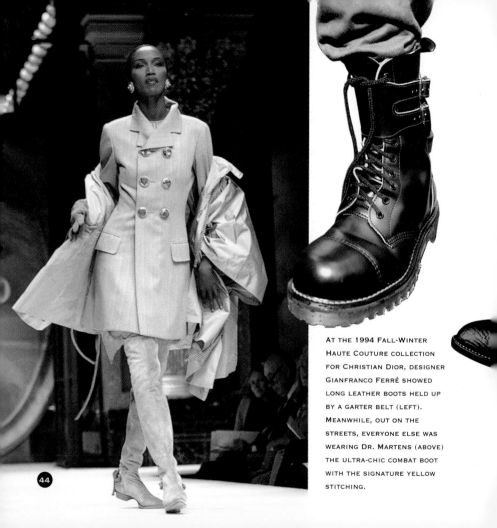

AT THE 1994 FALL-WINTER HAUTE COUTURE COLLECTION FOR CHRISTIAN DIOR, DESIGNER GIANFRANCO FERRÉ SHOWED LONG LEATHER BOOTS HELD UP BY A GARTER BELT (LEFT). MEANWHILE, OUT ON THE STREETS, EVERYONE ELSE WAS WEARING DR. MARTENS (ABOVE) THE ULTRA-CHIC COMBAT BOOT WITH THE SIGNATURE YELLOW STITCHING.

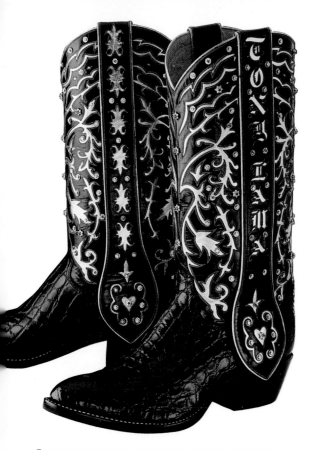

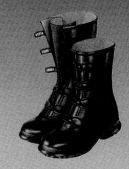

FOR THOSE WHO WANT TO DIE WITH THEIR BOOTS ON, A PAIR OF TONY LAMA JEWEL-ENCRUSTED ALLIGATOR COWBOY BOOTS CAN BE YOURS FOR ONLY $35,000 (PLUS TAX).

MEN'S BEST QUALITY EXTRA HEAVY WEIGHT ARCTICS MADE WITH THE FINEST GRADE RUBBER, REINFORCED, LEAK-TESTED AND WELDED, SOLD IN THE MONTGOMERY WARD CATALOG FOR $6.15 IN 1952.

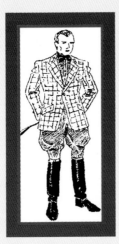

Tailors, bootmakers and hatmakers alike
know that men and women will never look as
good as they do in their riding gear.

Diana Vreeland

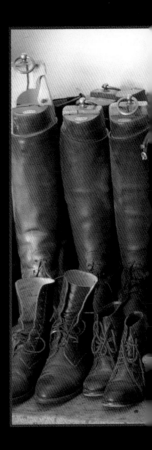

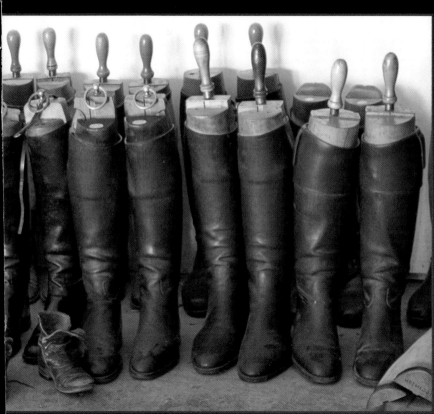

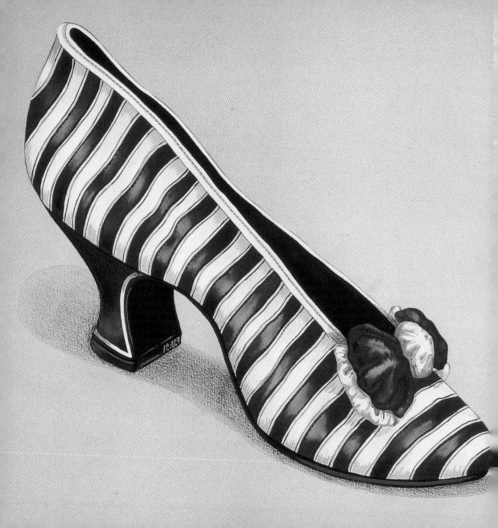

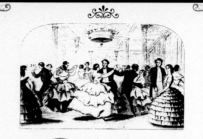

*H*ow far away the ball already seemed!
Why should there be such a distance between yesterday
morning and tonight? Her trip to Vaubyessard had made a
gap in her life like one of those great crevices that a storm
sometimes carves out in the mountains in a single night.
She resigned herself, however; reverently she packed away in
the chest of drawers her lovely dress and even her
satin slippers, whose soles had yellowed from the floor wax.
Her heart was like them; the wealth had rubbed off on her,
something that would never be erased.

Gustave Flaubert
Madame Bovary

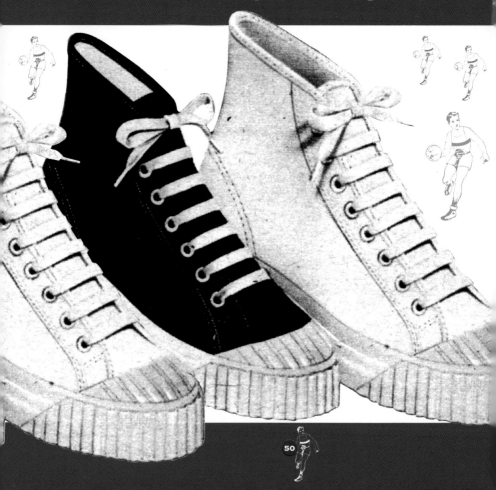

50

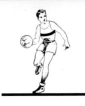

The bleachers were filled up with new basketball shoes. The shoes seemed blindingly, tragically white, as fresh as wet paint. The smell of shoes lifted straight from their boxes filled Ben's nostrils. A sadness gripped him as he realized how many pairs of new shoes were bought for nothing. The bleachers in this moment were ruled by virgin shoes and wool socks fresh from cellophane. The bleachers swarmed with youth unanchored, unpraised, and convulsed with the dreams of gangly boys and fat boys who wanted to be a part of something with a desperation that was almost palpable and alive.

The U.S. Market for basketball shoes amounts to **$407,000,000** a year.

THE NEW YORK TIMES
2/12/95

Pat Conroy
The Great Santini

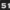

SHOESTORE STORE SHOE

In *Picasso: An Intimate Portrait*, Picasso's secretary, Jaime Sabartés, recalled that between 1939 and 1940, while passing a certain shoemaker on their customary walk in Royan, Picasso would invariably stop and comment on the same pair of shoes.

PICASSO: There's nothing extraordinary about that pair of shoes but somehow or other I like them. One of these days I'm going to go in and see if they fit me....

SABARTÉS: Why not now?

PICASSO: I'm not in a hurry. Let it go for some day when we get out a little earlier. You know I don't need them right away.

SABARTÉS: As long as they appeal to you what harm would there be in asking?

PICASSO: Of course there would be some harm! If we went in it would take a lot of time. They'd start a conversation, and then every time we went by we'd have to greet them. You know I don't mind this; but after two or three months we'd get to be friends, and then I'd have to worry about the health of the grandfather, the father, the baby ... and on top of it all I'd have to take the shoes.

Picasso was married when his soon-to-be-next-wife, Françoise Gilot, first noticed him in a restaurant.

We were still at table when Picasso and his friends left. It was a cool evening and he put on a heavy mackinaw and a beret. Dora Maar was wearing a fur coat with square shoulders and shoes of a type many girls wore during the Occupation, when leather, along with so many other things was scarce. They had thick wooden soles and high heels. With those high heels, the padded shoulders, and her hieratic carriage, she seemed a majestic Amazon, towering a full head over the man in the hip-length mackinaw and the *béret basque*.

Françoise Gilot
Life with Picasso

THE FEET WERE ALL WRONG . . . WITH A SORT OF WRONGNESS THAT HE FELT RATHER THAN KNEW. . . . IT WAS LIKE WEAKNESS IN A GOOD WOMAN, OR BLOOD ON SATIN; ONE OF THOSE TERRIBLE INCONGRUITIES THAT SHAKE LITTLE THINGS IN THE BACK OF THE BRAIN. HE WORE NO SHOES, BUT, INSTEAD, A SORT OF HALF MOCCASIN, POINTED, THOUGH, LIKE THE SHOES THEY WORE IN THE FOURTEENTH CENTURY, AND WITH THE LITTLE ENDS CURLING UP. THEY WERE A DARKISH BROWN AND HIS TOES SEEMED TO FILL THEM TO THE END. . . . THEY WERE UNUTTERABLY TERRIBLE. . . .

F. SCOTT FITZGERALD
THIS SIDE OF PARADISE

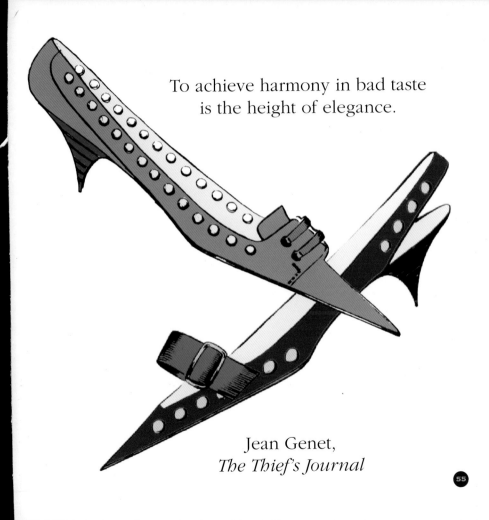

To achieve harmony in bad taste
is the height of elegance.

Jean Genet,
The Thief's Journal

"All the shoes that fit we print."

Today, rain, don't wear suede.
Tonight, cold, wear extra socks.
Tomorrow, you're on your own.

The Shoe York Times

Vol. XTRA   No. 8.5   ©1995 The Shoe York Times   *65 CENTS*

Many Mules for Marcos

Hidden slippers reveal softer side of dictator's wife

MANILA, March 29— In what has been described as the biggest cache of size six shoes ever amassed, Imelda Marcos, wife of the deposed president Ferdinand Marcos, inadvertently left behind more than 3,000 pairs (totaling 6,000 shoes) when she and Ferdinand fled the Philippines in a big hurry. Not knowing what to do with so many shoes, the government announced today that the collection would continue to be warehoused in the basement of the Malacana Palace where they are the sole responsibility of a worker named Tito Boniface Santiago. Due to the dank and musty storage conditions, the shoes require perpetual polishing.

Santiago reports that by the time he is finished polishing every pair, "it's time to start over." Meanwhile, the ousted dictatoress remains silent *(continued on page D5)*

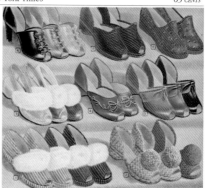

Risking his life and that of his family, janitor Santiago used a hidden camera to photograph these never-before-seen slippers, recently discovered in Imelda's guest bedroom.

(continued on page D5)

OBITUARY

Shoeman Dies at 105

Hector Teegordon, 105, died today in his home in Lowell, Massachusetts. Teegordon founded his company on the invention of the rubber heel. A former printer, Teegordon used to stand on a rubber mat to ease his tired feet as he set type. He grew weary of carrying the mat everywhere, and when his wife complained of skid marks on her flannel sheets, Teegordon nailed pieces of rubber to the heels of his shoes. Eventually, he patented the invention. Mr. Teegordon left his entire fortune to the *Save the Ferrets Foundation,* claiming his family deserved nothing. "They're just a bunch of loafers!" he wrote in his pithy Last Will and Testament.

Wedding Announcement

THE POCONOS, Sept. 8th— Solemates Countess Mitzi Von Ostermiller and tennis pro Skip Buckingham were married yesterday in an afternoon ceremony at the Chapel of Love Motor Lodge. The bride wore silver Chanel sling-backs with ankle bows from the *Printemps/Eté* 1994 collection. The bridegroom wore nothing of importance.

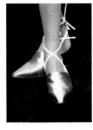

Footloose and Fancy-Free Foot Facts
by William Saffron

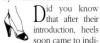

Did you know that after their introduction, heels soon came to indicate the status of the wearer by their height? Well, it's true. Rich people started wearing really high heels so that they could stand above the poor and that's the origin of the expression

well-heeled.

Originally, if you were called a **square**, it referred to the fact that you wore square-toed shoes long after they were out of fashion.

When used in combination, **well-heeled square**, the phrase describes a wealthy, but badly dressed person, or a country western singer.

Khrushchev's Shoe on Display

NEW YORK, October 4th — Nikita Khrushchev's famous shoe which he used to pound on the desk during an angry exchange at the United Nations General Assembly in October, 1960, has returned to

RUSSIAN WINGTIP CIRCA 1958

New York for a 35th anniversary celebration of the Russian temper tantrum heard round the world. The wingtip, part of a traveling shoe show, will be on display at the Thom McAnn Museum of Art through February.

A VOYAGE TO
≈ Lilliput ≈

For above seventy moons past, there have been two struggling parties in the empire, under the names of *Tramecksan* and *Slamecksan*, from the high and low heels on their shoes, by which they distinguish themselves.

It is alleged indeed, that the high heels are most agreeable to our ancient constitution: but however this be, his Majesty hath determined to make use of only low heels in the administration of the government and all offices in the gift of the crown, as you cannot but observe; and particularly, that his Majesty's imperial heels are lower at least by a *drurr* than any of his court; (*drurr* is a measure about the fourteenth part of an inch). The animosities between these two parties run so high, that they will neither eat nor drink, nor talk with each other. We compute *Tramecksan*, or High-Heels, to exceed us in number; but the power is wholly on our side. We apprehend his Imperial Highness, the heir to the crown, to have some tendency towards High-Heels; at least we can plainly discover one of his heels higher than the other, which gives him a hobble in his gait.

Jonathan Swift, *Gulliver's Travels*, 1726

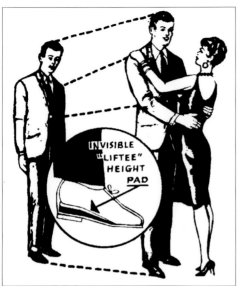

INVISIBLE "LIFTEE" HEIGHT PAD

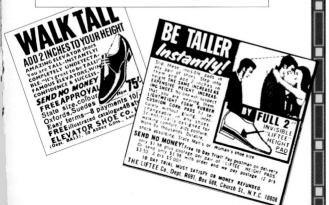

WALK TALL
ADD 2 INCHES TO YOUR HEIGHT
AMAZING ELEVATOR shoes
you are TALL INSTANTLY!
COMPLETELY UNDETECTA-
BLE. "It's great to be TALL"
FAMOUS ELEVATORS WIN
CONFIDENCE & SUCCESS.
SEND NO MONEY
FREE APPROVAL
State size, colour.....from 75'-
Oxfords, Suedes 10/-
Easy terms—8 payments
FREE illustrated catalogue4B st
ELEVATOR SHOE CO., Lon
(Dept. BA33), 50 Abbey Gdns., Lon

BE TALLER
Instantly!
Slip these invisible pads in
and pair of shoes. Step into
them and add 2 inches to
your height. THE same INCREASE
IN THE shoes No one will suspect
EXPENSIVE HEIGHT INCREAS-
ING SHOES. No one will suspect
that you are wearing suspect
LIGHTWEIGHT foam & them
CUSHION CORK PADS fit se-
curely without gluing. Inter-
changeable in any shoes.
Scientifically designed for
walking comfort, also good for
aids thousands. Durable.
Worn by thousands. Durable.
shock absorbing State Man's or Woman's shoe size
SEND NO MONEY! Free 10 Day Trial! Pay postman on delivery
only $1.98 plus postage per pair of "LIFTEE" HEIGHT PADS.
Or send only $1.98 with order and we pay postage. (2 prs
$3.50 3 prs $5.00)
10 DAY TRIAL MUST SATISFY OR MONEY REFUNDED.
THE LIFTEE Co., Dept. R691, Box 608, Church St., N.Y.C. 10008

In Greek tragedy, gods and heroes wore platforms to elevate themselves above the rest of the cast.

Egyptians wore them to raise their feet off the burning sand.

In Renaissance Venice, high society wore chopines to raise themselves above the water.

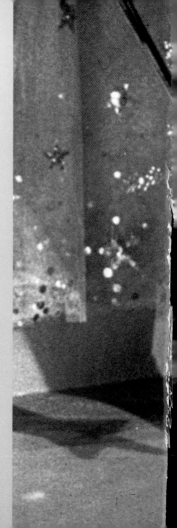

All you have to
do is to knock the
heels together three
times and command
the shoes to carry
you wherever you
wish to go.

Frank L. Baum
The Wizard of Oz

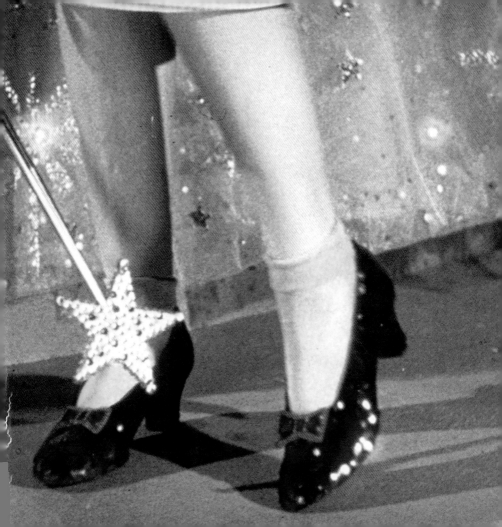

SPECIAL THANKS TO

Mary Kalamaras,

Emily Chewning,

Diana Catherines,

Bobby Griffin,

Denny Levy,

Nicole Mills,

Helene Cadario,

and Dolores Lusitania.

AND, OF COURSE,

Lena Tabori,

Hiro Clark,

and Hubert.

PHOTOGRAPHY AND ART

AP/Wide World Photos, 20.

Chanel, 57 (top left). Photo © Xavier Raoux.

David Cook, 1, 2, 3, 7, 18, 19, 39, 42 (right), 43. NOTE: the highheeled red toe shoes on page 39 were designed by Byron Lars for a Broadway Cares/Equity Fights AIDS celebrity auction, sponsored by *Mirabella* magazine.

Culver Pictures, Inc., 8.

Christian Dior, 44 (far right). Photo: © Frederic De Lafosse.

Dr. Martens, 44 (right).

Salvatore Ferragamo, 5, 10, 11, 15, 40, 41, 64.

Fratelli Rossetti, 4.

Virginia Halstead, 30-31.

Stephanie Hoppen Picture Archive Limited. Fiona Saunders satin shoe painting circa 1890, 48.

Samuele Mazza. The three shoes on the bottom of page 23 and one on 42 (far left) are part of an exhibition organized by Samuele Mazza, who invited artists to create shoe-inspired works of art. Featured on page 23, left: *Dinamica* (Dynamic) by Savitransport; center: *Ambivalenza* (Ambivalance) by Maurizio Dori; right: *She sells sea shells on the sea shore* by Shaun Clarkson. Page 42 (far left): *In vino veritas* by Giuseppe Arcofora. All shoes are featured in the book *Cinderella's Revenge* by Samuele Mazza (Chronicle). Reprinted with permission of Samuele Mazza and Idea Books.

Kit Latham, 47.

Tony Lama, 45 (left).

Libby Reid, 16-17.

Alexandra Stonehill, 36. Emilia's Slippers © 1992 by Alexandra Stonehill.

Tim-Street Porter, 23 (top right).

Mary Tiegreen, 24-25, 26, 52.

Turner Entertainment, 60. *The Wizard of Oz* © 1939 Turner Entertainment Co. All Rights Reserved.

Mario Valentino Int'l Inc., 23 (top left).

EDITORIAL

Brown shoes
don't make it.

Frank Zappa

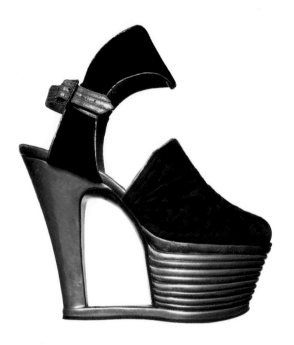

BEAUTY IS A SIMPLE PASSION,
BUT, OH MY FRIENDS, IN THE END
YOU WILL DANCE THE FIRE DANCE IN IRON SHOES.

FROM SNOW WHITE & THE SEVEN DWARFS

The End